# PERFECT SEX

## A succinct guide with lots of insight on how to derive maximum sexual pleasures

**ROSELYN DOUGLAS**

# TABLE OF CONTENT

# CHAPTER ONE

## WHAT IS BLOW JOB

A blow process is an act with the aid of which characters puts or insert their lover's penis of their mouth, and thereby, proceeds to suck and lick it for the man's preferred satisfaction. It's additionally called oral intercourse, fellatio, or instead, "happening on" someone. The female model is called cunnilingus.

# CHAPTER TWO

## HOW TO IGNITE BLOW JOB CONFIDENCE IN YOUR PARTNER

whilst you are in an extreme idea approximately the handiest ways that to give an awesome blow job in your guy, you will be inquisitive concerning these absolutely distinct fellatio positions and fellatio techniques nevertheless as some of a whole lot of advanced stuff like giving your man deep throat. However, there's a capture:

None of this facts is beneficial if you're acting first-rate awkward and fearful once you offer your man fellatio. A comparable is genuine once it comes all of the way all the way down to what intercourse positions you operate.

It will be an incredible deal a whole lot of sexually pleasing for your husband if you appear assured and grasp what you're doing.

If you're now not sexually confident, then this will be pretty study for you. Underneath are some exceptional fellatio guidelines that you just have to use to assist building your sexual self belief.

First-rate exercise:

If you want to get self belief inside the urge at the chance of taking place on your guy and studying a way to provide a smart blow process, then you definitely desire to take a look at 1st. but not basically for your guy. The best method is by using a vibrator or by means of putt a prophylactic device on companion diploma unpeeled, sleek banana.

Simply use warning to now not push the dildo/banana too so much down your throat to stop choking.

Building up sexual confidence:

It will be complicated listening to any individual bring up sexual self-assurance once making a try to fulfill your man. Being sexually assured isn't concerning being smart at intercourse. As a substitute, it's regarding being at ease in conjunction with your frame. They've even accomplished research that displays that the softer you are together with your body, they may be sexually happy every you and your husband are going to be.

So in case, you think that gaining knowledge of everything there may be to grasp on a way to gives a clever blow task goes to offer you all of the sexual self-belief you would love, then you're lamentably missing an essential purpose. To result in sexual self-assurance, you would like to set off comfortable with United Nations employer you are. The fact is that nobody is right, and everybody has things concerning themselves that they need to have been completely one-of-a-kind; however, it cannot be changed.

Men will be extraordinarily apprehensive:

Don't neglect that guys usually lack sexual confidence

conjointly. He is likewise disturbed regarding no longer obtaining an erection or possibly regarding dropping his erection and his erectile organ going soft. He conjointly is also disturbed concerning Cumming too quickly or not Cumming the least bit. Those are the principal matters that guys get apprehensive about, however, they may be lots greater.

So the following time you offer head in your guy, take into account essentially that he can usually be too disturbed concerning his own performance to be aware of any errors or awkwardness.

# CHAPTER THREE

## HOW TO MAKE HIM STAY WITH YOU

Every girl must understand the language of every man. Sure all guys have their sex languages but until you are capable of decode that truth, then I bet he'll need to stay with you for lifestyles, no matter any facet chick. Provide him time to determine out alternatives after you have got handled him based totally on few steps I've mentioned beneath, if study carefully and accompanied each commands given.

## THE FELLATIO FOREPLAY:

It can be beautiful to concentrate to, but, men love intercourse sports to be drawn out considerably longer pretty maximum ladies assume. So, whereas giving him a quickie BJ is superb warm for every of you (like say concealed away for a few minutes at a party), you'll realize that a slow, teasing increase goes to lead to your guy processing an even bigger load, and a fair larger smile on his face. This is regularly maximum probably the most powerful, but conjointly the most unmarked blow activity tip you'll be able to study. With this in mind, here rectangular degree a gaggle of pleasant "fellatio foreplay" hints which you really will use earlier than giving your man head:

Hand rubdown – This one is perhaps the simplest to urge right. Whereas you are hugging him, reproof him or while you're just bodily on the point of him, area your hand on his crotch. For this reason your hands have to be resting on his briefs or his trousers. To shape it sleek, begin with the aid of 1st putting your hand on his leg and transferring it up from there. Then sincerely softly start massaging his member and testicles outdoor of his trousers/briefs.

It's as honest as softly running your hands over this space, but, you will be capable of conjointly get a piece additional aggressive through softly grabbing and compressing his cock and balls and so cathartic the strain

After massaging him for a few minutes, facilitate him kick off his trousers and briefs. Then definitely hold doing what you have been doing, going for walks your palms over his manhood. in case you want, you will moreover softly trace your palms up and down his dick and round his balls. If you wish to discover extra jacking off techniques, then certify to observe out the jacking off component here.

Speak to Him on your Knees every other excellent blow activity tip to make up to giving your guy head is speech your guy while in your knees. You will kick off with one factor honest like, "So what does one want Maine to try to presently, baby?"

As you turn out to be extra assured and spot his enthusiasm, you'll begin increasing your grimy speaking, with the aid of

Telling him what amount you're playing giving him head.

That you genuinely can't wait to style his liquid frame substance.

But, giving him a blow process turns you on.

Of route, you'll talk grimy in the course of your blow process too. Communicate grimy also, it can help train everything you would like to grasp concerning intercourse.

So close – any other blow job tip you will do to make up for your blow task is to parent around his manhood initial. Therefore as opposed to virtually taking him into your mouth and giving him a blow process, you can:

Kiss round his crotch and groin.

Lightly massage his balls exploitation your tongue.

Softly "tickle" his testicles with the pointers of your hands.

The Kiss direction – A sandwich blow process tip that enables you to maneuver swimmingly from caressing your husband to taking him on your mouth is to determine slowly down from his lips to his phallus via caressing your way down. Therefore you may pass from his lips to his neck to his chest to his stomach until you attain his groin area. Of path, this works way better if he's naked.


## FLICK THE FRENULUM:

For lots guys, the most touchy spot on their phallus is their frenulum. The frenulum is that the face of the end in their phallus, anywhere the physical shape joins his shaft.

An intensely enjoyable blow activity tip that you in reality will use on him is to use the top of your tongue to use a sensitive flicking motion thereto. While you're clearly about to stimulate his frenulum while suction him (learn recommendations approximately suction here and right here) or honestly licking his phallus (analyze a few sexual perversion licking strategies here), this approach is absolutely one of a kind as you will be focusing all your stimulation on a truly particular purpose on his phallus.

Bear in mind that if your man has been circumcised, there may be an opportunity that his frenulum has been eliminated.

## SEVERE KISS:

Every other proper manner to start off your blow activity is through excessive kissing of his cock everywhere. Kissing is first-class if you wish to take matters slowly and teasing your guy.

You could kiss his phallus any manner you wish, but it'll be a great deal simpler once you operate your hand to carry it in situ while you kiss it. There rectangular degree more than one opportunity ways to kiss his phallus, from giving him little, fast 'pecks', to giving him longer, lots of severe kisses. He'll specially like it if you offer him similarly wet, sloppy kisses. Don't be shocked if you may be able to see precum or seminal fluid dripping from his cock at this degree.

Kissing him perhaps a gorgeous way in pulling returned, in case you're feeling him obtaining on the brink of climaxing and want him to have a hint longer earlier than accomplishing coming. It'll offer your jaw a relaxation if you discover it obtaining worn-out from having him on your mouth.

## SENSITIVE WITH ENAMEL:

You already skill touchy your boyfriend's member is, especially the face of head (aka the glans). For pleasuring it, that is often without a doubt a first rate factor…however in case you apply an excessive amount of strain, otherwise you square degree too difficult with it, and you they're progressing to hurt your guy. It's identical in your erectile organ and canal in case you're masturbating or your guy is going down on you. without a doubt believe however sore it is probably if your beau had nails that have been continuously catching on you…or worse, are you capable of consider however painful it might be if he began victimization his enamel on you as he changed into licking you out and playacting head. It is probably agony!

The best vital blow task tip once giving your man sexual perversion is that you simply completely have to not use your teeth on him. It will absolutely wreck accomplice degree in any other case extremely good BJ. But what if he's significantly nicely endowed or you have got little mouth?

In things like this, it is regularly actually not possible to avoid your enamel as you are taking him into your mouth. The primary issue you'll do is to wrap your lips round your teeth just so your lips act as a gentle barrier. the second one factor is specializing in techniques anywhere you don't take him into your mouth like these ones or with the aid of giving him a hand process facet notice: there's a little proportion of guys that get pride from it after you operate your enamel and observe a small little bit of pressure on his member, victimization associate degree truly feather light bit on him. My candid advices are doing now not try this till your guy feels the urge for it and mention it himself.

BLOWING HIM:

Many girls are for that reason traumatic at the notion of giving head to their guy, that they simply get instantly to that with very little or no construct-up and without a teasing. It's like they're targeted entirely on creating him ejaculate and obtaining that spermatozoa out of him. Lightly teasing your man and building up the sexual anxiety, so he's a good deal mendicancy you to blow him is important if you want to require your blow jobs from smart to high-quality.

One good manner to amp up the sexual tension and have the wiggly in satisfaction is to lick him gently, ensuring to use infinite spit and so blow at the wet patch you've created. Processing on a wet patch creates a cooling sensation that's excellent for teasing your man and creating him moan with satisfaction.

Attempt doing this for a couple of minutes before you are taking him into your mouth.

# CHAPTER FOUR

## INFLUENCE IN GIVING BLOW JOB

You run no risk of obtaining HIV so long as you do now not get any sperm cell in your mouth when you rectangular degree giving a blow job. But, you may nevertheless get STIs. Maintain smart oral hygiene. If you provide blow jobs at the same time as now not a contraceptive device, certify you commonly moreover get tested for STIs for your mouth.

Dangers in phrases of Sexual Transmitted infection (STIs):

While giving blow jobs, you run a risk of acquiring Cupid's disease, gonorrhea, Chlamydia or serum hepatitis for your mouth or throat.

An equal is proper the opposite method round: you will get partner STI if acquire a blow process from someone international health agency has Cupid's ailment, social disease or Chlamydia in his mouth or throat.

The longer someone offers you a blow process, the larger your opportunities of obtaining partner STI if he has one.

Cast off in addition hazard:

•	in case you would really like to provide blow jobs at the same time as not walking any hazard of HIV, certify you do now not get any sperm cellular on your mouth which the within of your mouth is not broken.

•	In case you are doing get sperm mobile to your mouth, do not swallow it however spit it out in actual-time. Then rinse your mouth sooner or later sedately and spit out the water.

•	keep clever oral hygiene and keep your tooth and gums healthful.

• Don't brush your tooth shortly earlier than or quickly whilst sexual perversion. This can prevent minor damage to your gums. Use the solution for latest breath or wait not less than an hour while brushing your teeth before giving a blow process.

• if you offer blow jobs at the same time as no longer a contraceptive tool, certify you typically moreover get tested for STIs in your mouth.

• if you would really like to scale back your opportunities of obtaining STIs and HIV the maximum quantity as manageable, use a contraceptive tool while you offer a blow task.

# THE END

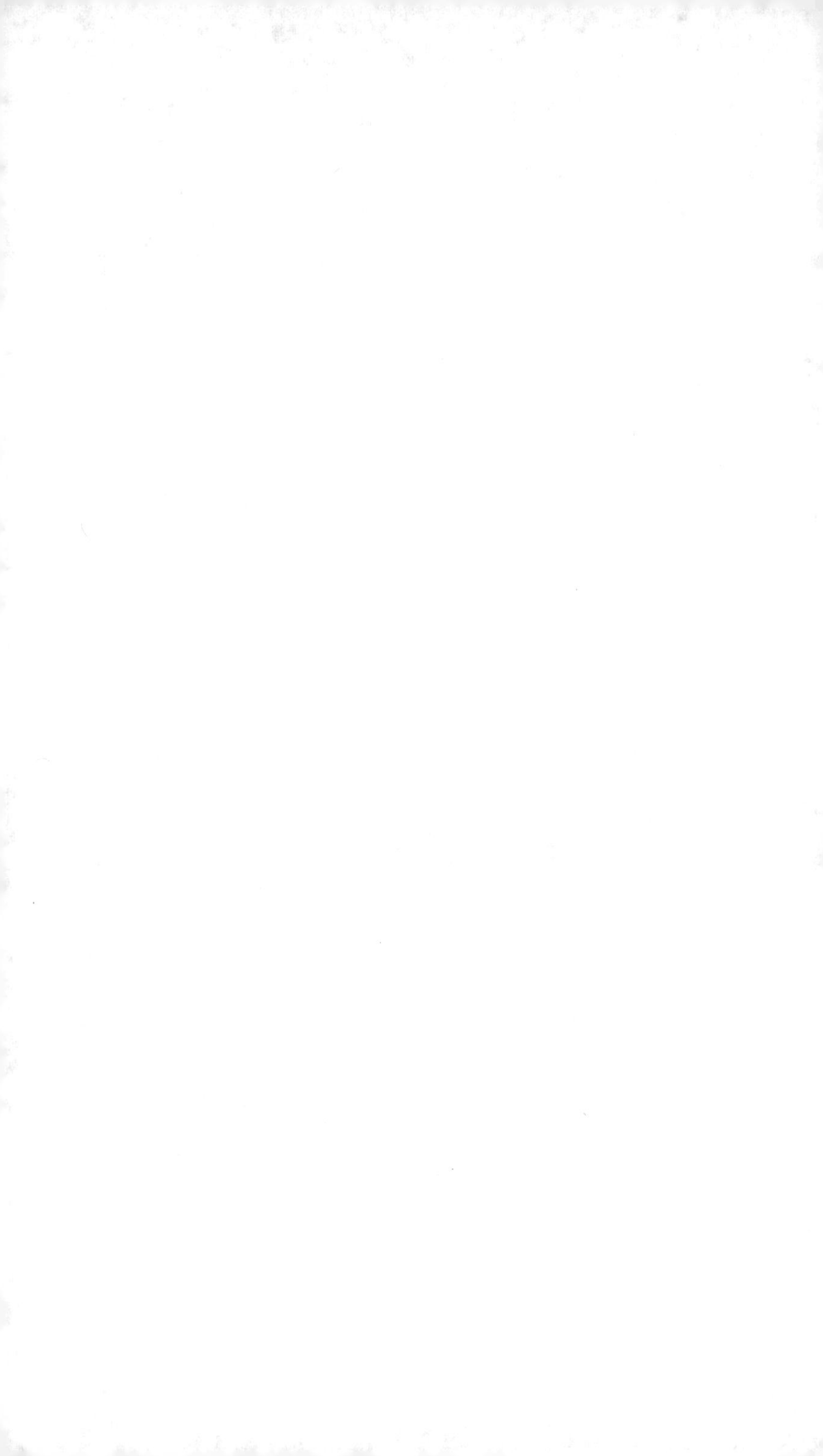